TRANSFORMING RELATIONSHIP THROUGH SEVEN TIME-TESTED PRINCIPLES

A GUIDE TO LASTING LOVE AND CONNECTION

By

Linda J. Lampley

Copyright

No part of this publication may be reproduced, distributed or transmitted in any form or by any means, including photocopying, recording or other electronic or mechanical means, except for the abbreviations contained in the main reviews and as permitted by law prohibiting third parties from publishing such contents.

Copyright © (Linda J. Lampley), (2024)

Disclaimer

The contents of this book, "Transforming Relationships with Seven Time-Tested Principles," are for reference purposes only. The information presented on these pages is based on research, experience and observations in the field of psychology.

While every effort has been made to ensure the accuracy and reliability of the information contained in this article, readers are advised to consult a professional or seek personalized advice appropriate to their particular circumstances.

The ideas, principles, and advice contained in this book may not be applicable to all relationships. Individual experiences, situations, and difficult relationships can vary greatly, and there is no one-size-fits-all solution.

Readers are encouraged to use their own judgement and discretion when following the instructions and procedures in this manual. The author and the publisher are not responsible for any consequences, damages or liabilities arising from the application or misinterpretation of the content of the publication herein.

It is important to remember that relationships are multifaceted and each partner's journey is unique. This guide is intended to provide guidance and insight, but is not a substitute for professional advice or treatment tailored to the individual's specific needs.

By reading and participating in the contents of this book, the reader acknowledges and agrees that the author and publisher are not responsible for any decisions taken or made based on the information contained herein.

Thank you for understanding and carefully reading the information presented in this book.

About the Author

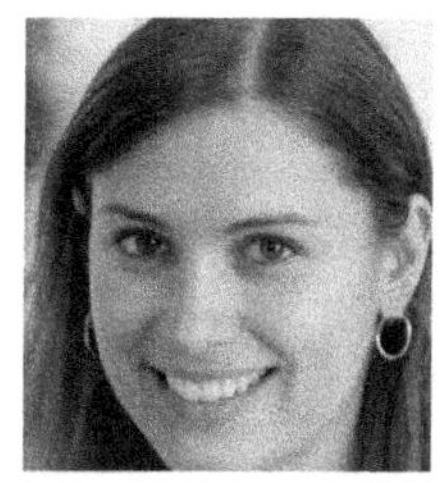 Linda J. Lampley is a beacon of insight and compassion in the field of social justice. She has a passion for developing and nurturing relationships and is an advocate for the development and success of partnerships.

As a writer, Linda is endowed with wisdom and insight that comes from her deep understanding of human emotions and interpersonal relationships. Her passion is helping people enjoy the best relationships and fostering connections that include understanding, respect and love. Episode Her passion for encouraging people to experience the joy of relationships is reflected in her advice and time-tested content.

Linda's work was published on the page. She joins his listeners to provide guidance and support to relationship seekers. Her dedication to encouraging fun and enjoyment in partnership is an inspiration that shines a light on long-lasting love and meaningful connections.

With her compassion and deep understanding, Linda J. Lampley embodies the essence of the Guide: an advocate for celebrating love, respect, and happiness in all relationships. Her work is a testament to his ongoing commitment to helping people build rich relationships and enjoy the joy that comes from meaningful, fulfilling relationships.

Table of Contents

INTRODUCTION

Marriage is a bond of communication between dreams, thoughts and desires, established on the basis of the principle that ensures the unity of two souls. A successful marriage essentially depends on the interplay of trust, communication, empathy and commitment. It goes beyond the shorthand meaning of passion and romance and has a deeper understanding, namely the bond that holds together the atmosphere in life.

The meaning of eternal marriage is not in big shows or happy moments, but in complying with the principles that support the relationship well. It is a fabric of mutual respect, unwavering support, and the ability to grow together despite life changes.

In our study of the seven principles, we understand the wisdom gained from many years of research and real-life experience. Once established and implemented, these principles become the foundation of a successful marriage.

Each principle is a building block in itself, paving the way for eternal love and creating a place where partners can grow, develop and find comfort in living with each other.

Join me on this journey as I share secrets, ideas and insights to nurture a marriage that will stand the test of time, the foundation of mutual understanding, inner harmony of relationship and unconditional commitment to keep love alive. the complexity of life.

CHAPTER 1

UNDERSTANDING FRIENDSHIP IN MARRIAGE

Are you and your accomplice experiencing difficulty making an association? Companionship in marriage is vital to foster love with your mate. In any case, sadly, now and then our connections experience because of occupied timetables or stress. This guide will show you how to work on your companionship and work on your relationship with your accomplice or accomplice.

What are the benefits of friendship education in marriage?

- **Increase Parental Happiness.** Research shows that having your partner as a good friend in your marriage can increase marital satisfaction. The benefits of companionate marriage are long-term and can lead to adulthood. Couples can increase their marital happiness by doing little things that bring joy to their relationship. Friendship provides an emotional bond that can lead to marital satisfaction.

- **Improve Communication** Marriage is a period when communication between spouses can cause problems. Good communication is the key to a successful marriage. Being a good listener can benefit your relationships with friends. Good listening can help provide clarity and prevent marital conflict.

- **Build emotional and physical relationships.** Relationships are built through conversations and sharing personal information. Relationships are built when you open yourself to other people and allow them into your life. The key to a good relationship is trust; You need to be comfortable with the other person before sharing this information. Relationships based on strong friendships are more successful. Relationships are supported by physical closeness and emotional closeness. Some of its benefits include increased communication, romance, physical intimacy, parenting, and sexual health.

- **Forgiving Your Bad Behaviors** Remembering your actions will help maintain peace in your relationship. But we are all human and making mistakes is part of our DNA. Always apologize and be honest when you make a mistake. Doing this shows that you are responsible for your actions and willing to correct mistakes. Having a friend in your marriage can help increase forgiveness in your relationship. Also, having someone to talk to and confide in can help you forgive your spouse.

- **Build trust in marriage** A good relationship with your partner helps build trust and respect. Friendship can help couples discover each other's personalities and interests and establish a healthy relationship. It also allows spouses to get through difficult times together. A healthy marriage is based on trust and respect. Couples who incorporate these qualities into their relationships will experience happiness and longevity.

HOW CAN YOU CREATE A SPECIAL INTIMACY WITH YOUR ACCOMPLICE?

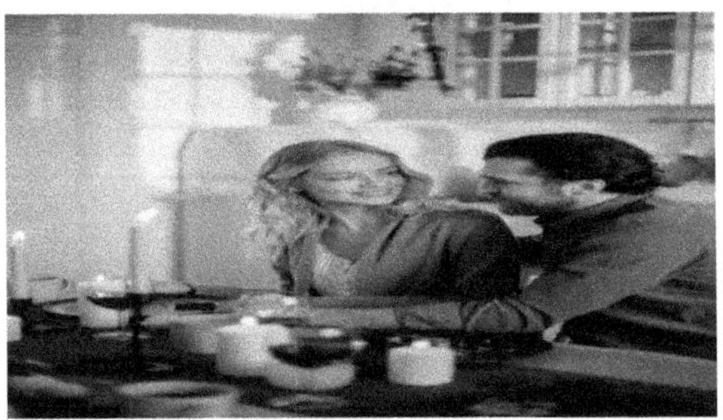

- **Spend time together**. To build a strong friendship with your spouse, spending time together is very important. We need to engage in common interests and discuss important issues. Play together and celebrate each other's uniqueness! Other ways to get to know each other include browsing, hanging out, and sharing interests.

- **Comprehend and communicate** in your accomplice's way to express affection. One of the most amazing ways of turning into your accomplice's closest companion is to learn and talk about their "essential way to express affection." We as a whole have various approaches to communicating and getting love; In our marriage, these needs are frequently not met. On the off chance that you can require some investment to figure out how your life partner says love and really try to address that issue, it will go far in revamping your companionship.

There are five essential main avenues for affection: acts of service, quality time, words of affirmation, gifts, acts of service, and physical contact. Sadly, we frequently expect our spouse to "know" what we need and assume that they know how we want to be loved. Regardless, this isn't overall the situation. Assume you're not sure what the person you're talking to says about their primary way of showing affection, and look for clues in their behavior. Additionally, the three questions listed below will help you pay attention to your answers. How could I at any point help you? How can you make your life easier? How can I be a good husband or wife?

- In marriage, we try to satisfy each other's feelings. It is likely that the most important thing you can do to further develop your family relationships is to understand and satisfy each other's most important feelings. Emotional needs are feelings that let us know that we are important, valuable, and loved by our partner. When these needs are met, we feel welcome and secure in the relationship. On the other hand, when we are ignored, we may feel ignored, unimportant, and unloved.

It is very important that everyone's emotions are unique. What is a requirement for one person may not be a requirement for another. This is why it is so important for your life partner to tell you what he wants from you. If you don't know what their needs are, ask them! It may seem awkward at first, but it will get easier with practice. And it will be worth it when you see the difference in your relationship.

- **Be present and prioritize your marriage**. Please prioritize marriage. It's not your job and it's not your colleagues'. The enemies of family harmony are workaholism and excessive ambition. Your partner needs to be in your physical presence and close to your home. Likewise, a man's masculinity can help keep his loved ones safe and supported. Likewise, your loved one needs respect and sexual satisfaction.

Zeroing out absolute sexual energy in a marriage eliminates the risk of extramarital affairs and social breakdown.

WHAT IF YOU AND YOUR PARTNER AREN'T FRIENDS?

Relationships are not designed to meet everyone's needs, and being good friends with your husband is good, but not essential. It's nice to have other good friends in your life.

A good friend can talk about anything, even things your husband doesn't like. Being friends with your spouse helps you have a healthy marriage. It is important to be honest with each other, even when it is difficult. Friendship should include the ability to confront difficult issues. Conflict may give way to growth. Compassionate marriage overcomes conflict.

How do you find time to make friends in your busy schedule?

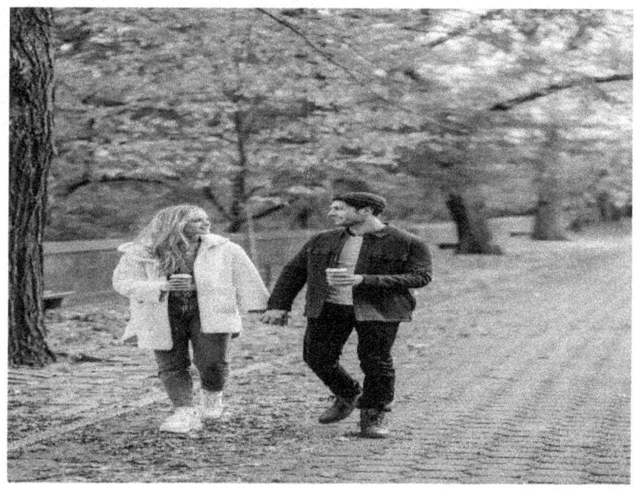

- Spend time together every week to build good friendships. Shows the challenges and advantages of being honest and communicating effectively.

- Play together, laugh often, and appreciate each other's differences.

- Celebrate your partner's successes (forget their failures).

- In a busy marriage, make time for friendship by accepting each other, letting each other be who they are, supporting each other, and being kind.
- Trust, responsibility and mutual respect are crucial to a good relationship; so stay focused and work on projects together.
- Learn how to act fairly so disagreements don't ruin your relationship.
- Conflict is a good time to strengthen friendship.
- Create daily rituals to help you stay close, including prayer and shared interests. willing to learn from each other and discuss simple topics.
- Talking often is one of the best ways to make time for companionship in a busy marriage.

Remember that you enjoy spending time with your friends and always make time for yourself. appreciates harmony in all aspects of your relationship, making time for friends.

CHAPTER 2

PRINCIPLE 1: CREATING LOVE MAPS

Creating a love map is like creating a detailed roadmap of your partner's inner world. This is about deepening your understanding of each other, developing empathy, and strengthening the emotional connection in your relationship.

Understanding Love Maps

Love map reflects your knowledge of your partner's likes and dislikes, dreams, fears, values, and everything else that shapes your personality.

It is a mental plan that develops over time as you learn and grow together.

Importance of Love Maps

- **Emotional Connection:** Strengthens intimacy and trust by laying the foundation for deep emotional connections.
- **Communication**. A well-developed love map improves communication by reducing misunderstandings and conflicts.

Steps to create a love map

- **Active Listening:** Practice active listening. Ask open-ended questions, show genuine interest, and listen carefully to your partner's thoughts and feelings.

- **Share experiences:** Share memories, stories, and experiences to deepen mutual understanding. This helps fill in the gaps in your love map.

- **Curiosity.** Be interested in your partner's evolving interests, goals, and aspirations. Encourage open dialogue about their life journey.

- **Regular check-ins:** Keep your love map up to date, checking in on each other's feelings and thoughts through regular conversations.

Exercises to strengthen your love map:

- **Question session.** Schedule regular sessions where you take turns asking each other questions to discover new aspects of your partner's life.

- **Share Memories:** Deepen your connection by sharing past experiences, childhood memories, and life stories.

- **Share your dreams:** Discuss your aspirations, dreams, and plans for the future to align perspective and understand each other's goals.

Creating a love map is a journey of discovery and connection. This is an ongoing process that requires effort, curiosity, and active participation. By investing time and energy into understanding your partner's world, you can develop a relationship based on mutual understanding, compassion, and love.

UNDERSTANDING THE PROBLEM OF EMOTIONAL DISCONNECTION DUE TO LACK OF KNOWLEDGE ABOUT EACH OTHER

Disagreements in relationships are often caused by a lack of understanding of each other's inner lives. When partners feel conflicted, it's often because they haven't explored each other's thoughts, feelings, and experiences. These misunderstandings can occur in a variety of ways.

Signs of conflicting thoughts.

- **The discussion is not over.** Discussions will be off-topic and lack depth and emotional resonance.

- **Discomfort**. Your partner may feel misunderstood or not truly felt, which can lead to confusion.

- **There is less intimacy.** Feeling separate can reduce physical and emotional intimacy.

- **Inconsistency**. At the same time, partners may feel distant from one another or as if they have less.

- **Misunderstandings**: Difficulty understanding each other's feelings and experiences.

Reasons for interfering with work.

- **Busy schedules** or distractions can limit opportunities for constructive discussion.

- **Thought**: Assuming you already know everything about your partner will hinder your desire to explore deeper.

- **A connection could not be established.** Lack of effective communication can lead to misunderstandings or avoidance of important conversations.

- **Overlooking self-improvement.** As planned, your partner will not understand these changes, so communication will have to stop.

Impact on Relationships

Emotional conflict can destroy the foundation of a relationship, resulting in loneliness, anger, or distrust. This impacts the emotional stability and relationships necessary for effective collaboration. Emotional conflict that arises from not understanding each other's inner feelings is a relationship problem. But by recognizing the signs, understanding the causes, and using strategies to deepen understanding and connection, partners can strengthen their relationship emotionally and creatively and achieve better relationships and greater satisfaction.

TECHNIQUES TO CONTINUALLY UPDATE AND DEEPEN KNOWLEDGE ABOUT YOUR PARTNER'S WORLD

Your relationship may change depending on the season, and in some cases, the cold season may be too cold to feel the warmth of spring. Sometimes reconnection is accompanied by persistent minor interruptions. Sometimes he waits for the burdensome task of snow removal to reveal life's additional complex stressors.

How, you inquire? You can begin by integrating the accompanying expressions into discussions with your accomplice. They will assist with keeping you tuned into one another inwardly, open the lines of correspondence and explore struggle in a useful manner.

- **Tell me more.** The phrase "tell me more" is as significant as "I love you." This expression is tied in with staying inquisitive about your accomplice while likewise being locked in with the things they're telling you, whether it's a paltry business day show or a serious problem. We begin to believe we know the other person and begin to lose the wonderful listening and attention we gave them earlier in the relationship, which is one of the main reasons relationships fail.

By rehearsing our tuning in — which is dependably about the other individual and not about us — we remind them we are still here, and we are reminded that they are likewise still here.

- **Something I'm battling with right currently is ...** Similarly, it's critical to summon interest inside yourself about your accomplice, letting them in on what's happening in your world is additionally significant. They need to be aware assuming you're feeling anxious working, self-basic, or sincerely depleted. Understanding what's going on inside you helps them practice more persistence and resist the temptation to literally think about it when you're feeling calm or in a bad mood."

- **"...is truly giving me pleasure at this moment "This** is an enhancement to the above question and is a method for breathing satisfaction into your relationship. " Feelings are infectious, so let your accomplice ride the energy of your positive sentiments. Likewise, suggestive association is stirred up by allowing your accomplice the opportunity to encounter you participated in what causes you to feel invigorated and energetic. Let your light sparkle. "

- **" How would you like to feel ...?** "**This** weekend, on your birthday, on this excursion. This minor departure from the " what is it that you need to do? " Question is tied in with studying what your accomplice needs to have and sustaining your affection toward them on a more profound level. For instance, to feel cherished, loose, and blissful on their birthday, even if you realize they aren't enthusiastic about consideration, then you know not to design a major birthday slam with everybody your accomplice knows.

- **" I'm attempting to figure out your perspective "Contentions** are essential for any heartfelt connection, and the manner in which you explore them can either carry you nearer to one another or make a wedge. Regardless of whether you concur with your accomplice's perspective, telling them you're attempting to comprehend can be amazing in gaining ground. " On the off chance that you truly mean this, it will take you quite far to see someone when it is languishing. We aren't intended to continuously concur, but it is generally essential to attempt to comprehend your accomplice as far as conceivable so you can compromise and feel upheld together. By overcoming difficult situations in a helpful way, it makes the future more charming on the grounds that you're better at exploring difficult situations due to effectively vanishing them previously.

- " **How might I appear to you this week? "Regardless** of whether you're in a crisp winter season, it's quite simple to slip into scorekeeping with your accomplice (for example, I stacked the dishwasher last time, or I awakened three evenings in succession with the child. The issue with this is the' how have you helped me of late?' attitude, which can raise disdain. "Assuming that the two accomplices turn the tables and the spotlight on' how have I helped you recently?' Then, at that point, everybody's needs are met, yet from the perspective of abundance as opposed to shortage. Ask it week by week, perhaps on a Sunday night as you get ready to move into another week. "

- **" It implied such a great amount to me when you..."** We are designed to search for what's up, says Solomon, so we benefit from rehearses that assist us with seeing the best in everyone around us. What we focus on, we get a greater amount of, so pointing out what you value will assist you with getting a greater amount of that. That practice of gratitude revitalizes personal relationships. " While much of this language can be used consistently in daily and weekly discussions, meeting in a space on a regular basis (even if scheduled) is not an entirely unrealistic idea.

Emotions, interests, and needs are constantly changing. So, intentionally connect with your partner in a trusting way so that you can feel a sense of unity, solve problems together, and remind each other how much you care about each other.

CHAPTER 3

PRINCIPLE 2: MAINTAINING AFFECTION AND RESPECT

Maintaining affection and respect involves intentionally creating a culture of gratitude and honor in your relationship.

Try these strategies to increase affection and respect in your relationship:

- **Practice gratitude every day.** Leave a glowing note expressing your appreciation for your accomplice's traits or actions. Verbal confirmation. You can express your admiration by constantly expressing sincere praise and gratitude.

- **Review positive memories. Think** about it together. Reminiscing and sharing precious moments or memories will bring you and your partner closer. Create new memories: Deepen your relationships by creating new positive experiences on a regular basis.

- **Recognize kindness in small actions and gestures**. Whether it's making an expression or giving a good hug, try paying attention and appreciating the details that you easily overlook.

- **Respect for development and flexibility.** Recognize Growth. Celebrate self-improvement and accomplishments by building on each other's progress and strengths. Supporting difficult times: Express your respect for your colleagues' solidarity and patience in difficult moments.

- **Focus on your qualities.** Recognize and communicate the strengths and special qualities of allies you admire.

- **Show interest in and dynamic commitment** Participate in their interests. Show genuine interest in your accomplice's leisure time or interests by participating in discussions and movements related to his or her interests.

- **Demonstration of awareness Shocking Act** Plan a shocking or kind act to show your gratitude and love.

- **Public Recognition**. Show respect or appreciation to your accomplice in public or among loved ones.

- **Embrace your weaknesses.** Share snapshots of weaknesses and shortcomings to foster deeper communication and understanding closer together.

- **Be proud and celebrate your uniqueness.** Accept and appreciate each other's uniqueness and contrasts, and remember them as an important part of your relationship.

Supporting attachment and respect involves making an intentional effort to consistently acknowledge, appreciate, and praise your partner's characteristics, activities, and developments. By using these different techniques, couples can develop a culture of gratitude that strengthens their bond and expands communication in new and authentic ways.

PROBLEMATIC DECLINE IN RESPECT AND AFFECTION

When respect and affection begin to wane in a relationship, it can be an anxious and difficult time. Here's a new way to solve this problem:

- **Think about personal change tolerance.** Take time to look at any personal changes or changes that may have affected your feelings of respect and affection.

- **Determining Relationship** Understand the Dynamics: Recognize changes in relationship dynamics that may be contributing to a decline in respect and affection.

- **Revisit your shared values.** Review and discuss shared values, aspirations, and goals to rekindle unity and connectedness.

- **Open and honest communication**. Engage in open conversations about changing emotions and express vulnerability without judgment.

- **Create new and meaningful moments.** Introduce new activities or experiences that provide shared fun and connection.

- **Invest in emotional intimacy.** Promote emotional intimacy by sharing your feelings and thoughts with each other openly.

- **Recognize effort and growth.** Recognize and celebrate each other's efforts and personal growth and encourage mutual respect and admiration.

- **Cultivate gratitude.** Make it a habit to express gratitude to each other every day for your presence and positive contributions.

- **Professional guidance.** Consider seeking the advice of a therapist or counselor to help You understand these changes and find solutions together.

- **Focus on the positive.** Intentionally focus on each other's positive qualities and strengths to create new feelings of admiration.

Confronting a decline in respect and love requires self-reflection, open communication, and active action to reignite the spark in your relationship. By engaging in personal reflection, fostering honest communication, investing in shared experiences, and seeking external guidance when needed, couples can work together to rebuild respect and affection and grow a stronger, more lasting bond.

STRATEGIES TO INCREASE INTERGRITY, APPRECIATION AND RESPECT IN EVERYDAY INTERACTIONS

Here are some effective strategies to help. You cultivate gratitude, gratitude, and admiration in your everyday interactions.

- **Express gratitude every day.** Start or end your day by verbally thanking your partner for something they do or simply for being in your life.
- **A sincere compliment** Throughout the day, give your partner sincere compliments about their qualities, actions, or efforts.
- **Thoughtful action.** Surprise your partner with small, thoughtful gestures like

cooking their favorite meal or leaving a heartfelt note.

- **Active listening.** Show genuine interest in your partner's thoughts and experiences by actively listening without distraction.

- **Gentle gestures.** Offer hugs, kisses, or gentle touches to show affection and appreciation throughout the day.

- **Recognize effort.** Recognize and appreciate the effort your partner puts into their daily tasks or responsibilities.

- **Share positive memories** Reminisce about happy moments. Remember shared positive experiences that spark feelings of admiration and gratitude.

- **Cultivate gratitude.** Make it a habit to express gratitude to each other every day for your presence and positive contributions.

- **Professional guidance** Consider seeking the advice of a therapist or counselor to help You understand these changes and find solutions together.

- **Regular Affirmations.** Start or end your day by affirming your love, respect, and gratitude for your partner, either verbally or through a written note.

- **Mutual Appreciation:** Encourage both partners to engage in actions and expressions of gratitude for one another.

Consistently incorporating these strategies into your daily interactions will develop a culture of gratitude, gratitude, and admiration in your relationships. By expressing gratitude, giving sincere compliments, making affectionate gestures, and acknowledging each other's efforts and accomplishments, partners can create an atmosphere of mutual admiration and gratitude in their everyday interaction.

CHAPTER 4

PRINCIPLE 3: TURNING TOWARDS EACH OTHER

Cheerful suggestions and enthusiastic attempts at mutual help increase the level of positivity during conflict discussions. The strongest relationships are built from the beginning. One of the biggest predictors of relationship success is the ability to turn toward each other, continually nurture the relationship, and make daily efforts to connect with your partner and accept offers of emotional connection. Most fights in relationships area result of rejecting and opposing these suggestions. Denial and opposition mean both suppressing negativity and being in attack-defense mode. Cheerful suggestions and enthusiastic attempts at mutual help increase the level of positivity during conflict discussions. It also helps you replenish your emotional bank account, maintain strong, healthy relationships, and rekindle your romance.

Here are simple and effective ways to build a deep and lasting emotional connection with your loved one and show your commitment and care throughout the day.

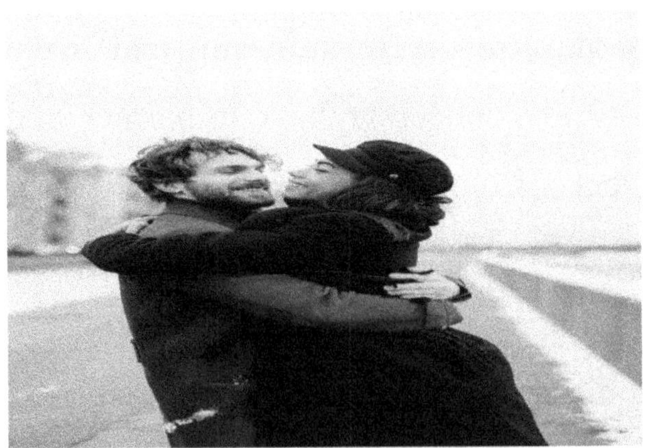

- Hug your partner in the morning and tell him how grateful you are to wake up next to him every day.
- Pay your full attention to your partner when he or she talks about work or family.
- Address the needs of your partners, big and small.
- A kiss hello and goodbye (a 6-second kiss is ideal and has romantic potential).
- Find out verbally when your partner seems nervous.
- Compliment with your partner.
- Join your partner when he or she does household chores.

IDENTIFYING ISSUES RELATED TO NEGATIVE EMOTIONS AND LACK OF OPPORTUNITIES

Uncertainty and lack of opportunity to connect are issues that slowly erode the fabric of relationships. Accepting these problems is important to heal and strengthen the mind.

Emotional Detachment

This problem manifests itself in many ways; It often occurs as a gradual decrease in emotions and connections between people. Symptoms of mental illness may include:

- **Poor Communication:** Communication decreases or becomes difficult, and meaningful conversations become scarce or absent.

- **Depression:** Loss of interest in common activities or interests that once provided joy and connection.

- **Too much distance:** Differences in emotions or feelings of difference, with the partner feeling distant despite being physically close.

- **Avoidance of Complaints:** Reluctance to open up and share feelings or concerns due to fear of judgement or rejection.

- **Lack of support:** Lack of motivation or understanding during difficult times leads to social isolation.

Busy Times for Connections

Missed times for deep connections are usually due to:

- **Idle Lifestyle:** Busy times and the important factor is the need to spend quality time together.

- **Poor Communication:** Inability to understand or respond to emotional instructions resulting in inconsistent timing.

- **Untapped Interests:** Ignoring opportunities to engage in common activities or hobbies that could strengthen a connection.

- **Assumptions and Expectations:** Unspoken expectations or assumptions about relationships That causes us to not have time to express our thoughts or needs.

Addressing conflicts of interest and lack of networking opportunities requires effort. This includes open communication, vulnerability, and a willingness to devote time and energy to building relationships. By recognizing these issues early, individuals and couples can take conscious steps to rebuild relationships, build relationships, and create a strong foundation for their relationships.

THE PRACTICE OF HAVING SIMILAR FEELINGS AND ACTIONS

Emotional investment in a relationship is the foundation of long-term connection. Developing and maintaining this deep feeling requires conscious practice and effort from both parties. Strategies for encouraging consistent work and building strong relationships are discussed below.

- **Give importance to open communication:** Open and honest communication is the basis of unity. Encourage an open conversation where both parties feel comfortable sharing their thoughts, fears, and desires without fear of judgement. Create an environment of empathy and understanding by listening to your communication partner's cues and responding effectively.

- **Embrace vulnerability:** Allow yourself and your partner to be vulnerable. Share your feelings, fears, and vulnerabilities openly to create a safe space for emotional relationships to flourish. This creates an environment of trust, acceptance and support, leading to emotional bonding.

- **Empathize:** Empathize by trying to understand your partner's feelings. Even if you don't understand how they feel, show genuine concern and support their feelings. Empathy strengthens relationships and strengthens emotions.

- **Good Time, carelessly:** Devote your good time regularly to deep relationships. Minimize distractions and engage in activities that encourage meaningful and collaborative conversations. Whether it's a quiet dinner together or a walk in nature, these moments can lead to an emotional connection.

- **Appreciate and Appreciate:** Express gratitude and appreciation for your partner's presence and contribution to the relationship. Regularly acknowledging and affirming each other's efforts and qualities strengthens the emotional bond and fosters a sense of value within the relationship.

- **Mutual Respect and Support:** Show respect for each other's opinions, boundaries, and aspirations. Offer unwavering support during both triumphs and challenges. This mutual respect and support deepen emotional trust and solidarity.

- **Adapt to Changing Needs:** Recognize that emotional needs may evolve over time. Enjoy these changes and be willing to adapt and grow together. Being flexible and willing to adapt to each other's emotional changes is key to maintaining a healthy relationship.

- **Periodic Evaluation and Treatment Process:** Continuously evaluates the emotional state of the relationship. Discuss what worked well and areas that need improvement. Willingness to change course and adjust to having a good relationship.

Regular application of these ideas creates space for emotional communication, thus strengthening the foundations of the relationship. By encouraging open communication, vulnerability, empathy, and mutual support, couples can create emotional connections that last into their relationships.

CHAPTER 5

PRINCIPLE 4: ALLOWING PARTNER'S INFLUENCE

Allowing your partner to influence you is an important part of a healthy, healthy relationship. This involves understanding each other's thoughts, preferences, and feelings and incorporating them into decision-making processes and everyday interactions.

Here's why and how your partner's personality can help your relationship.

- **Social justice and equity:** Convergence in educational decision making. Respect your partner's thoughts and feelings. This promotes equality in the relationship and recognizes the importance of both parties' opinions.

- **Share your solution.** Shared decision-making encourages collaboration. Evaluating and integrating ideas creates shared ownership of choices and creates strong commitment and satisfaction with the results. Improve communication.

- **Allow your injured partner to encourage open and honest communication.** This creates an environment where both sides are heard and respected, which leads to deeper understanding and connection.

- **Building trust.** When partners put in the effort, trust and confidence in the relationship grow. It signals a willingness to work together to improve relationships and promote stability and hope.

- **Respect differences.** Partners often have different thoughts, values, and interests.

Allowing for influence means finding a middle ground in building relationships that acknowledge differences and respect each other's individuality.

DYNAMICS OF THE BALANCE OF POWER

This prevents exclusivity or dominance in the relationship. Instead, it promotes a balance of power, ensures equality, and encourages growth and direction in relationships.

- **Harness the power of your partners.** Listen carefully. Pay attention to your partner's feelings and don't ignore them. Respect other people's thoughts and feelings, even if they are different from your own.

- **Compromise and Compromise:** The willingness to compromise and find a solution that takes into account the perspectives of both sides. Flexibility in decision-making allows you to find ways to meet your partner's needs.

- **Discussion and debate:** Be open to discussion when making decisions. Discussions that take into account different perspectives aim to find common ground that takes into account the interests of both sides.

- **Effective Results:** Build effective partnerships by recognizing, valuing, and involving each partner in the decision-making process.

By allowing one partner to influence the other, couples can build a relationship of harmony and harmony based on intimacy, shared decision-making, and a deeper understanding of each other's needs.

PROBLEM OF POWER STRUGGLE AND LACK OF COMPROMISE

Disagreement and conflict can damage relationships and lead to anger and communication problems. These problems and their solutions are described below.

- **Battle for Control:** Struggle often stems from a need for control, respect, different expectations, or judgement. This happens when one or both parties try to control the relationship or the stress.

- **Conflict:** Conflict occurs when one or both parties are unwilling to express or evaluate another point of view.

- **There is no middle ground:** If your partner refuses to change or refuses to make decisions or solve problems, it will be difficult to find ground.

Address power issues and open dialogue

Initiate patient and respectful dialogue to address the underlying issues that lead to power conflicts. Encourage open discussion so you can understand each other's feelings and concerns without criticism or judgement.

- **Find the problem:** Determine the cause of the explosion. Understanding these benefits can help you avoid or prevent stressful situations.
- **Use your knowledge and understanding.** Be sensitive to your partner's thoughts and feelings. Understand their needs and motivations and try to understand their problems.
- **Compromise Agreement:** Both parties must be willing to compromise. Focus on

finding a solution that works for both parties, based on compromise and respect for each other's needs.

- **Improve your communication skills.** Improve your communication skills by listening, accepting and solving problems. Learning how to express your thoughts and feelings can help reduce resistance.

- **Professional help.** If you need the help of a counselor or therapist, The Outsider can provide information and guidance on strategies to resolve and reconcile your issues with power.

- **Set Common Goals:** Work together to set common goals for your relationship. Shared goals build relationships by encouraging cooperation and harmony.

Resolving conflicts of power and influence requires cooperation from both parties. By encouraging open communication, mediation, compromise, and asking for help, couples can resolve these issues, build trust, and improve their health, cleanliness, and sociability.

CHAPTER 6

PRINCIPLE 5: SOLVING SOLVABLE PROBLEMS

Resolving solvable problems in relationships with solutions that have clear solutions and can be managed effectively through mutual understanding, communication and compromise. Here are the steps to follow to resolve such issues:

- **Report the issue:** State the issue without pointing fingers. Focus on specific situations or behaviors that cause anxiety. Express your feelings:
- **Use the word "I"** when expressing your thoughts and concerns to avoid appearing

negative. Explain how the issue affects you personally.

- **Brainstorming solutions:** Collaborating to create solutions. Encourage creativity and openness to find options that meet the needs of both parties.

- **Evaluate solutions together.** Consider the pros and cons of each idea and its potential to solve the problem.

- **Consensus and Compromise:** Choose a solution that suits both parties' perspectives. Aim to reach a compromise that satisfies and respects both parties.

- **Implement solutions:** Provide suggested solutions for action. Commitment follows a plan to solve problems effectively.

- **Evaluation and Adjustment:** Regularly review the results of the solution. Adjust or change if necessary to ensure success.

Example scenario:

Let's assume the problem is related to home operation. A partner may feel overwhelmed by work and need more help. Both parties discuss and agree on a joint family plan. They assigned specific tasks, agreed on a fair distribution, and set aside a week to discuss desired changes. Problem solving involves collaboration and problem solving that emphasizes compromise, effective communication, and willingness to compromise. By following these steps, couples can effectively solve these problems and strengthen their relationship by working together to find a good solution.

INABILITY TO HANDLE EVERYDAY CONFLICTS EFFECTIVELY

What is Conflict?

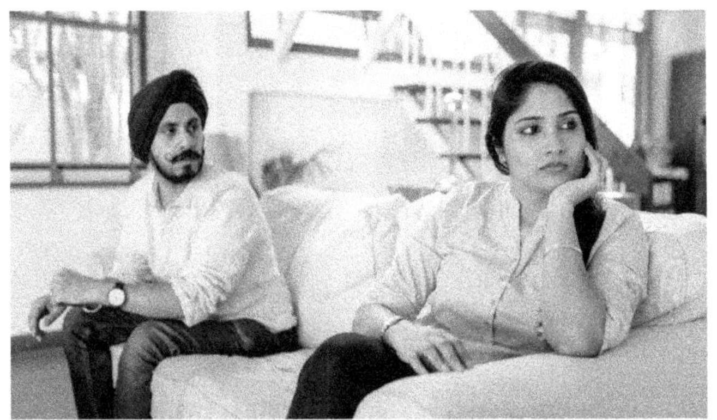

Conflict can be seen in every relationship. After all, you can't always expect two people to take the lead. It's important to learn how to deal with problems rather than fearing them and avoiding them. Conflict can be detrimental to a relationship if not handled properly, but when approached with respect, conflict provides an opportunity to strengthen the right relationship between two people. Learning these skills can help you bridge the gap in your healthy life and build better, more productive relationships.

- **A conflict is something other than a dispute.** This is what happens when one or two players see danger (real or not). If this is ignored, the conflict will continue to escalate. Because conflict is perceived as a threat to our well-being and survival, it will stay with us until we face it and resolve it.

- **We react to conflict based on our impressions** of the situation rather than an intensive examination of the current reality. Our understanding is influenced by our history, culture, values and beliefs.

- **Conflict evokes strong emotions.** You cannot resolve a conflict if you are dissatisfied with your own behavior or if you are unable to control your emotions.

- **Conflict is a time to grow.** Trust is built when you are willing to handle difficult situations in a relationship. It may be comforting to realize that your relationship may be full of stress and conflict.

Causes of conflict in a relationship

Conflicts arise due to differences big and small. This happens when people disagree about values, motivations, feelings, emotions, or desires. Sometimes these differences may seem minor, but when conflict leads to strong emotions, personal needs are often the root of the problem. These needs range from the need to feel safe, secure, respected, and valued to the need to feel connected and connected.

Consider the needs of children and parents. A child's need is to explore, so going outside or going to the edge of a cliff can satisfy this need. However, parents' desire to ensure their children's safety can only be achieved by limiting exploration. Conflict arises because these demands are incompatible. The needs of each party play an important role in long-term relationships.

Everyone deserves respect and attention. Failure to understand different needs in a relationship can led to distancing, arguments, and separation. Different demands at work can result in harm, reduced benefits, and unemployment. Recognizing conflicting needs and being willing to resolve them with compassion and understanding can help you solve problems, build teams, and build relationships.

How do you respond to conflict?

Are you afraid of conflict or do you run away from it? If your perception of conflict is based on painful memories from childhood or past negative relationships, you may think that all conflict ends badly. You may feel contradictions such as hatred, shame, and fear. Conflict can be destructive if experiences early in life leave you feeling weak or out of control. If you are afraid of conflict, it can turn into personal success. When you're already in a threatening conflict situation, it can be difficult to resolve the issue in a healthy way. Instead, you are more likely to be calm or angry.

Conflict resolution, stress, and emotions

Conflict can be emotionally draining and lead to anxiety, depression, and discomfort. If done poorly, it can lead to conflict, resentment and breakdown. However, when conflict is resolved in a healthy way, it helps you understand other people, build trust, and strengthen your relationship. If you are out of your thoughts or too anxious and can only focus on certain thoughts, you cannot understand your own needs. This will make it difficult for you to communicate with others and determine what is really bothering you. For example, couples often argue about small differences (the way he hung his towel, the way he ate his soup) rather than the things that upset them.

The ability to successfully resolve conflict depends on your ability to:

Regulate pressure quickly, remain alert and calm. By remaining calm, you can accurately review and record verbal and nonverbal communication.

Control your emotions and behavior. The moment you take charge of your own emotions, you can express your needs without undermining, threatening, or rejecting others.

Pay attention to what other people say and how they feel. Know and embrace contrasts. Problems are often resolved more quickly if you refrain from lewd words and actions.

Nonverbal communication and compromise

When people argue, the words they use rarely convey the essence of the issue. However, paying close attention to the other person's non-verbal signals or 'body language' - facial expressions, posture, gestures, and tone of voice - can help you better understand what the other person is actually saying. This allows us to respond in a way that promotes trust and focuses on the real issues. Emotional awareness is essential to our ability to accurately understand others. The more you pay attention to your own emotions, the easier it will be to pick up on the quiet signals that reveal other people's emotions. While you're struggling, think about what message you're sending to others and whether what you say matches your nonverbal communication. When you say "I'm okay" and grit your teeth and look away, your body is clearly showing you that you're not okay. An interested look, a gentle touch, and a calm voice can all help ease the tension in a conversation.

More methods for overseeing and settling struggle

You can guarantee that the most common way of overseeing and settling struggle is just about as sure as conceivable by adhering to the accompanying rules:

- Tune in for what is felt as well as said. At the point when you truly tune in, you associate all the more profoundly to your own requirements and feelings, and those of others. Listening likewise reinforces, illuminates, and makes it more straightforward so that others could hear you when it's your chance to talk.

- Make compromise instead of winning or "being correct." Keeping up with and fortifying the relationship, instead of "winning" the contention, ought to continuously be your main goal. Consider other people's opinion. Focus on the present. Holding on to resentment from past conflicts will limit your ability to face the reality of your current situation. Instead of focusing on the past and admitting guilt, focus on what you can do in the present time and place to solve the problem.

- Pick your battles. Conflicts can be draining, so it's important to consider whether the problem is actually worth a significant investment. You might not want to give up your parking space if you've been spinning in circles for 15 minutes, but there are so many parking spaces that arguing over one spot isn't worth the effort. sorry.

- Conflicts cannot be resolved if you are unwilling or unable to forgive others. The only way to change the situation is to give up the desire to punish. This only makes life complicated and tiring.

- Know when to let something go. If you can't reach an agreement, declare a ceasefire. It takes two people to resolve a dispute. If the disagreement cannot be resolved, you may decline to participate and continue.

Use Humor to Compromise Through Smart Communication

You can avoid many fights and resolve disagreements and conflicts. Humor can help you make statements that are difficult to convey without criticizing someone. But in reality, you should be giggling with the other person rather than at them. When we use humor and play to reduce tension and anger, reframe issues, and put things in perspective, arguments can truly be transformed into opportunities for more meaningful communication and intimacy.

MAKING LIFE DREAMS COMES TRUE

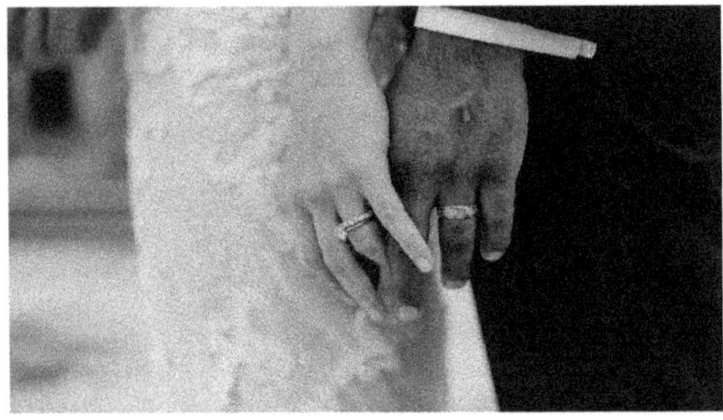

When building a house, you must start from the foundation. The foundation of Home Health Relationships is friendship. It creates a solid core consensus and facilitates conflict management. When conflict is managed well, you can focus on creating harmony and making a house a home.

According to statistics, couples who improve their skills in all areas of Home Health are more likely to have happier, more satisfying relationships over the life of the relationship. Think of the "House of Relationships" as a time that represents the couple's ability to strengthen the present (through friendship), eliminate the past (through control of conflict), and invest in the future (through creativity and dreams).

Once you've decided to commit, there's no reason to delay investing in the future. Start by learning what it means to achieve the dreams in your life. In short, this may mean spending more time on marriage matters than on weddings. Many women (and a few men) have dreamed of their wedding since childhood. This checks out. I said dream, dream big.

Your wedding should be a perfect representation of the hope, beauty, trust and love you want in your relationship. After all - remember, it's just a day - the wedding is still just a representation. a symbol

Symbols are dangerous because they only convey meaning. We all know that some people's houses are big, beautiful, a symbol of success and happiness, with a sea view. You might even call them "dream houses." These couples will never be able to realize their dreams together.

The house is symbolic but not the reality of the real relationship. I don't steal nice houses. I want someone so bad. I'm just saying that symbols must match reality in order for you to create meaning in your relationship. What if your dream house is first and foremost your dream house? But what if the real question in your home is "What if?" Well, the real answer to this question is "Let's make it happen!" whereas? Couples who can dream and pursue their dreams together are the ones whose neighbors are always jealous.

The first step is to know what your dream is. In primary school, "What do you want to be when you grow up?" Do you remember your answer to the question? What was first? Now? I asked: What do you want to do when you grow up?

Think bigger than your business. Where do you want to go? What do you really want to achieve? Which issue do you wish to resolve? Which mountain might you want to ascend? Which legend could you need to meet? Which book would you like to peruse? Which book would you like to compose? What do you want your children to tell you on your 50th anniversary? What would you like to write on your gravestone?

Could you at any point address these inquiries? Does your partner have one? The second step to achieving your dream life is to find out what your dream life is. If you don't know your partner's answer, find out. You may find that some dreams are very simple. "I've always wanted a sports car." It can, and doing so is an investment in the future. Make it a habit to daydream out loud and immediately check things off your list. One of my dreams is to remember my childhood with my partner. This is what I should have done.

My partner and I went to where I grew up and met some of our old friends and neighbors, laughing, crying, and reminiscing. This is a blessed from heaven. Not because I need to cross something off my list, but because I need to do it with my partner. This is a great gift for our family.

What is your dream? What do they represent? For me, this visit isn't about visiting my old neighbors, it's a reminder of where I was and where I am now - it also reminds me of a childhood dream. Your dream shows not only what you want to be, but also who you want to be.

When you think about the future, who do you want to be and what do you want to do? Not as a person, but as a couple. You can decide together which is the best way to build your relationship in the home of your dreams.

Could you at any point address these inquiries? Does your partner have one? The second step to achieving your dream life is to find out what your dream life is. If you don't know your partner's answer, find out. You may find that some dreams are very simple. "I have for a long time truly needed a game vehicle. It can, and doing so is an investment in the future. Make it a habit to daydream out loud and immediately check things off your list. One of my dreams is to remember my childhood with my partner. I ought to have done this.

My partner and I went to where I grew up and met some of our old friends and neighbors, laughing, crying, and reminiscing. This is a blessed from heaven. Not because I need to cross something off my list, but because I need to do it with my partner. This is a great gift for our family.

What is your dream? What do they represent? For me, this visit isn't about visiting my old neighbors, it's a reminder of where I was and where I am now - it also reminds me of a childhood dream. Your dream shows not only what you want to be, but also who you want to be.

When you think about the future, who do you want to be and what do you want to do? Not as a person, but as a couple. You can decide together which is the best way to build your relationship in the home of your dreams.

CHAPTER 7

PRINCIPLE 6: OVERCOMING GRIDLOCK IN CONFLICTS

Resolving relationship conflict requires a balance of patience, empathy, and open communication. Downtime can be unpleasant when a partner is at a disadvantage, but it also provides opportunities for growth and understanding. This is one way to describe how to overcome difficulties.

In relationships, it often happens that two paths diverge, which leads to stagnation, a type of conflict. At a fraught time, both sides find themselves in the midst of opposing views that will test the foundation of their relationship. Harmonious understanding suddenly ceased, emotions took over and words became useless. The root of this distrust is deep faith. They don't need help or, conversely, they need recognition and recognition. This turns into a war where compromise is impossible and the desire to understand is replaced by the desire to listen. But hidden within this uncertainty is the potential for radical change. Partners urged to approach the conflict not as enemies but as friends seeking understanding. They need to stop, step back, take a deep breath, and think about the thoughts that are causing this dissatisfaction.

Communication bridges the gap between different perspectives. This bridge is built by carefully choosing the words to express your feelings and listening carefully without interrupting others. This is an interactive process in which both parties interact with each other's thoughts and feelings, even if they have completely different views.

To overcome problems, we must find a foundation, a common place where unity and values live. This is where partners begin to discover the hidden treasures of shared goals and dreams, and remind themselves that their relationship is built on a solid foundation.

Change is needed. The will to bend without breaking. As professionals, it is the art of compromise that allows partners to respect both sides' views and find solutions, however imperfect, that are harmonious enough to bridge the gap. Patience can help during difficult times.

It is about understanding that solutions do not appear immediately, but emerge as a result of evolution and continuous effort. They realize that when they approach conflict with understanding and compassion, it contains the seeds of growth and deepening.

Sometimes wisdom sees morality as a sign of hope. A consultant or mediator acts as a guide, illuminating the way forward and providing tools to navigate the seas of conflict.

Ultimately, navigating conflict within conflict is a beautiful dance. The interplay of emotion, communication, and resilience. It is a collaborative journey exploring the vision of understanding the issues of conflict and harmony between different musical genres. Resolving relationship conflict can have a transformative effect. This can help partners move beyond the awkwardness of confrontation toward deeper understanding and a stronger bond.

EXAMPLE SCENERIES OF OVERCOMING GRIDLOCK IN CONFLICTS

Here are some hypothetical scenarios that show ways to handle conflict in a conflict situation:

Scenario 1: Parenting Style Conflict Sarah and Mike find themselves in conflict over parenting. Sarah believes in a more disciplined approach to parenting, while Mike prefers a more tolerant, liberal approach.

Overcoming conflict:

They decided to have a disagreement to resolve the issue. Both shared their concerns and the importance of being a distraction-free parent. Sarah shares her thoughts on the importance of setting standards and boundaries. Mike emphasizes the need for freedom and creativity in parenting. When they listen to each other, they achieve one goal: to make their children healthy and happy. They seek harmony; They create a balance that combines structure and free content. They agree to set clear boundaries while giving children the space to express themselves within these boundaries. They solve problems and develop shared parenting strategies by finding common ground in common goals.

Scenario 2: Disagreement over financial priorities

Emily and Alex have a disagreement over financial priorities. Emily values saving for the future and significant long-term financial security. In contrast, Alex believes in enjoying the moment and spending more money on spontaneous experiences and recreational activities.

Overcoming the Impasse: Realizing the impasse, they made an appointment for a financial meeting. Everyone expresses their own opinion and accepts the validity of other people's opinions. While Emily emphasizes the importance of financial security, Alex emphasizes the importance of enjoying life right now. In their conversations, they share their common values of enjoying life together while building their future. They create a plan that allocates a portion of their budget to savings and investments, while also allocating necessary funds for experiences and entertainment. They broke the ice by aligning their financial priorities with their shared values and created a plan based on their shared values.

Scenario 3: Different perspectives on work

Jenny and Chris face problems at work. While Jenny wants to be someone safe and important to move up the corporate ladder, Chris dreams of finding entrepreneurship and embracing risk and innovation.

Overcoming conflict:

After understanding the dilemma, they engage in open dialogue to explore their desires more deeply. Jenny and Chris talk endlessly about their career goals and the reasons behind their choices. Through dialogue, they share a common goal of personal success and success. They seek a compromise; They look for a way to provide stability that will allow Chris to slowly pursue his business dreams, while Jenny begins to manage her business. They decided to re-evaluate and support each other as they continued their journey. Recognizing their shared success, they broke the ice and created a plan that would fulfill both their desires

HOW TO HANDLE YOUR SPOUSE BAD HABITS

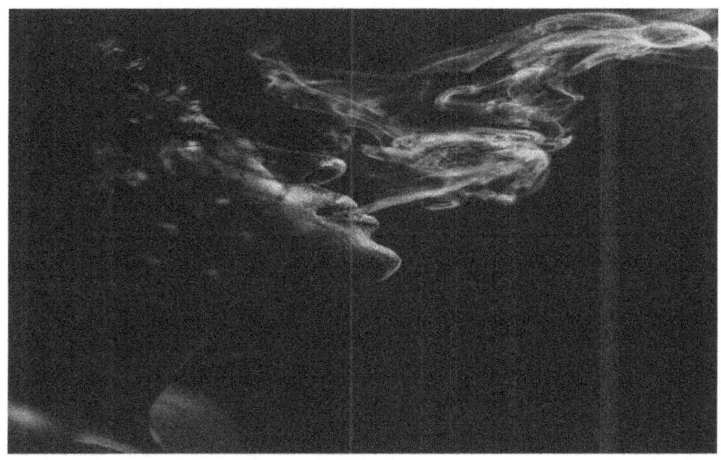

A spouse who drinks too much, eats too much, or smokes can do more harm than good to his or her own health. Doing this could also harm your partner. We worry about our loved ones and it is very difficult to watch them self-destruct with the risks of various diseases. But the definition of bad behavior is delicate. How can we be efficient in the process and help our partners? In this article, we will try to answer these questions and give you some tips on what to do and not to deal with your spouse's bad behavior.

- **Get involved**, don't criticize If your partner eats or drinks too much after work, don't argue, find something to do together. Find something to keep them from drinking again. Consider going to a park or visiting a museum. Be sure to find activities that you both enjoy and keep your partner away from ways that will encourage bad behavior.

- **Don't compare your spouse to others.** One of the things that upsets you the most is starting to start comparing. Don't compare your partner to others, try to make them feel good about their abilities or how their health would be if they worked harder to break something bad. If you focus on their potential, they will most likely start to open up to you about their inner pain. When you criticize and compare, you don't open up the conversation and cause your partner to hide their feelings even more.

- **Do not associate with other family members.** This attack is just embarrassing and usually not a good motivation. Your partner may also feel betrayed that you are now sharing what's going on in your personal life with others without their permission. If you want to have an "uncomfortable" conversation, make sure you don't involve others, as this will only damage your relationship with your partner. It may be tempting to have others support you, but most of the time you know when someone has a bad attitude. There is no need for anyone else to provide evidence.

Are you worried that your spouse's bad behavior will ruin your relationship? Contact a professional to find out what you can do to help your partner without making him or her feel like you don't put his or her best interests first.

CHAPTER 8

PRINCIPLE 7: CREATING SHARED MEANING

Creating shared meaning in complex types of relationships is the foundation of stable connections. This includes shared values, dreams, and goals that form the foundation of the couple's relationship. However, when these shared meanings are absent or unclear, problems can arise that affect the foundation of the relationship.

Meaning of unification.

Share meaning that promotes unity and purpose in your relationships. It is an invisible thread that runs through everyday interactions, guiding the couple through the twists and turns of their lives. It includes shared values, beliefs and life goals and provides a sense of direction and unity.

Problems related to lack of shared meaning.

- **Perception of conflict:** A lack of shared meaning can lead to conflict between partners. Without a shared vision, couples can feel disconnected or misunderstood.

- **Conflict and Conflict:** Conflict occurs when partners have different goals or objectives. Visual conflict can cause long-term negativity, making it difficult to find your footing.

- **Lack of direction:** Without common goals, couples find it difficult to live together. Without a clear path, uncertainty and multiple paths to the future can arise.

- **Emotional disconnection**: A lack of shared meaning can lead to emotional conflict, which makes it difficult for partners to understand each other's experiences and feelings.

PATHWAYS TO CULTIVATE SHARED MEANING

- **Open Communication:** Have an open and honest conversation about values, dreams, and aspirations. Discuss what is most important to each other and how they may or may not be different.

- **Collaboration:** Create moments of collaboration and memory. Participate in activities that encourage connection and build unity.

- **Create common goals:** Set common goals that concern both parties. Whether it's career aspirations, family plans, or personal growth, identify mutual objectives to work towards.

- **Value Appreciation:** Acknowledge and appreciate each other's values and beliefs, even if they differ. Cultivate respect for each other's perspectives.

- **Seek Guidance Together:** Consider seeking guidance from a therapist or counselor to navigate through differing values and align perspectives constructively.

In relationships, shared meaning serves as the compass that guides partners through the intricacies of life. It is a tissue woven from common values, dreams and goals that nourishes the sense of belonging and purpose. Addressing the lack of shared meaning requires an effort to understand, reconcile, and create a common vision for the future. By creating shared content, couples can strengthen their bond and pave the way for a harmonious and harmonious relationship.

CHAPTER 9

THE MOST IMPORTANT THINGS IN MARRIAGE

Marriage rate has diminished lately. While there are many reasons for this, it is clear that many people still want to get married. However, the number of long-term marriages is decreasing. Every couple is different and their relationships are also different. Therefore, there is no single magic formula that will make you happy forever. But there are some important points for a long term, healthy partnership. Here are three most important things in marriage:

- **Commitment**: Commitment is more than the desire to stay together for a long time.

It is the act of choosing a partner in life and being determine to overcome all the ups and downs together. Marriage when there are plenty of fish in the sea means that you are committed to making the relationship last and eliminate the doubt that this is just a temporary experiment

- **Love**: While most couples begin their relationship with love, maintaining their feelings for each other requires effort, sacrifice and sincerity. True love means putting your partner first and giving yourself without expecting anything in return. It also helps you accept each other as they are, flaws and all, and forgive each other when you fall out.

- **Respect**: If both parties in marriage do not respect each other, love, no matter how sincere, will have little meaning.

Respecting your partner's qualities, opinions and abilities means you not only accept but appreciate your differences. Respect also helps you listen to each other and work through problems and disagreements.

Of course, although these are the most important factors in marriage, there are many other factors that contribute to a happy marriage, such as patience, communication, relationships, high trust, sensuality and fun.

WHAT ARE THE MOST COMMON PROBLEMS IN MARRIAGE?

No matter how happy your marriage is, you are bound to encounter problems, big and small. One of the secrets to a healthy relationship is understanding potential problems and working to overcome them. Some common problems in marriage are:

- Lack of trust
- Lack of communication
- Jealousy and rivalry
- Financial problems
- Parental problems
- Difference of opinion

A vexing problem, especially in the context of injustice, is lack of trust. Faith is perhaps one of the most important foundations of marriage. So how can you increase trust in your relationship?

How to build trust in a marriage.

They say trust is more fragile than glass and can be broken with a single blow. And once lost, it is difficult to regain. Have confidence in your marriage. Keep the promises you make, no matter how few. Show up for your accomplice when he really wants you. Communicate your thoughts sincerely and straightforwardly. Stay calm and tell them they can trust you. Be patient and listen.

Sometimes, despite your best efforts, marriage can still be difficult to manage. However, with commitment, love, respect and trust, you and your partner can get through even the most difficult times. If it's all mistakes. Don't hesitate to seek the help of a relationship counselor whenever you need it.

CHAPTER 10

THE IMPACT OF TRUST AND COMMITMENT

As in all other human relationships, commitment in marriage is an important part of the relationship. Trust is the basis for building love and respect. As long as there is commitment, it is possible for marriage to withstand life's greatest challenges. Marriage is a deep-rooted responsibility for two individuals to cherish and uphold one another. Putting the needs of others before your own and working to solve their problems is a commitment.

Essential Elements of Marital Commitment

- **Communication** One of the most important aspects of marital commitment is good communication. Couples can share their needs, feelings, and thoughts by communicating. Additionally, communication enables partners to work together to solve problems in the relationship.

Forgiveness: We must understand that no one is perfect and everyone makes mistakes. For your relationship to last long, you need to be able to forgive your partner when he makes a mistake. It also helps to ask for forgiveness when you make a mistake. Forgiveness is a powerful tool in a relationship and is crucial to the success of your marriage.

Trust: Another important element of the marriage contract is trust. Trust is the basis of relationships. Without trust, relationships are lost. Trust is worked over the long run through genuineness, correspondence, and an eagerness to be open and powerless.

- **Sacrifice and Compromise** Responsibility in marriage likewise requires penance and split the difference. Marriage is difficult and at times one accomplice might need to forfeit for the other.

- **Making time for each other**: Time spent alone is one of the most important aspects of marriage commitment. It's important to spend time with each other, spend quality time together, and work to keep the spark in your relationship alive. Couples can do this through date nights, weekends, or traveling together.

WHAT HAPPENS WHEN THERE IS A LACK OF COMMITMENT IN MARRIAGE?

It is important to remember that neither partner will have a contract. Therefore, it is important that both partners understand their commitments and communicate openly and honestly with each other about any concerns or issues.

Lack of commitment in marriage can lead to the following problems.

Lack of communication: A common problem is the need for more communication. For example, let's say one partner is not committed to the relationship. In this case, they need to invest more to ensure that communication lines are open and problems are resolved quickly and efficiently.

Infidelity: Another problem that can arise from a lack of commitment is dishonesty. If a partner is not committed to the marriage, they may be more likely to cheat or be unfaithful. This can cause significant pain and suffering to others and lead to the destruction of trust.

Lack of intimacy and physical affection: Lack of commitment can also cause parents to fail to fulfill their desires in their marriage, such as a lack of intimacy and physical affection. For example, let's say one partner is not committed to the relationship. In this case, they will not make much effort to maintain physical contact with their partner. This can hinder romantic love and lead to divorce.

Feeling unappreciated or neglected: In some cases, a lack of commitment can leave the partner dissatisfied and unsupported. For example, let's say one partner isn't trying to make the relationship work. In this case, other people may think that they are not valuable or valuable.

Divorce: In the worst-case scenario, lack of commitment can lead to the end of the marriage. These problems can be solved if the problems caused by lack of commitment are solved. However, this may cause the couple to decide to end their marriage.

It is important to remember that marriage is a journey and commitment is an ongoing endeavor, not a final one. Therefore, when consensus cannot be reached, problems must be solved and resolved together.

WAYS TO IMPROVE COMMITMENT IN MARRIAGE

The decision to get married is a process that takes time and requires constant effort and attention. It can't be accomplished for the time being yet rather an excursion that requires persistence and devotion.

The following methods can help you make your partner more committed to you.

Setting shared goals: One way to increase commitment in your marriage is to set goals and work together to achieve them. Shared goals can be anything from money to personal development or even travel goals. Working together can strengthen the relationship between two parents and make them feel better.

Be on the same page with your partner: One more method for reinforcing responsibility in your marriage is to ensure you are in total agreement with regards to pursuing significant choices. This means talking openly and honestly about your values, beliefs, and goals, and agreeing with them. Working together will help prevent future misunderstandings and conflicts. Showing love and affection to your partner is very important. You can do this through small actions, like writing a letter, buying a small gift, or cooking your favorite meal. This small act of kindness can have a big impact on your relationship.

Make constant effort: One of the most important things to remember when it comes to wedding vows is that it's a two-way street. Both parties must be willing to put in the effort and make a commitment to each other. This means being willing to get along, help each other, and support each other through the ups and downs of life. The importance of people cannot be overemphasized. Imagine life without a partner.

Seek professional help: It's important to ask for help when you need it to maintain commitment in your relationship. It helps if you don't wait until your marriage is on the verge of ending before seeking help. That would be too late. Asking for help when needed can help prevent problems from escalating and provide insight and ideas to solve problems. Professional help can come from counselling, therapy, or talking to a trusted friend or family member.

Commitment in marriage is essential to the success of a relationship. Trust is the basis for building love and respect. Communication requires forgiveness, sacrifice and compromise.

They also need to make time for each other and keep the spark in the relationship alive.

CHAPTER 11

SUSTAINING GROWTH AND CHANGE

The seeds of growth in an intimate relationship are planted in the partners' shared experiences, desires, and common interests. Encouraging change and growth in a relationship is not just a place, it is an ongoing journey; a commitment to adapt, change and evolve together.

As life expands, relationships in relationships also expand. Change is not just an option, it is a social necessity. It means being willing to work through the challenges and changes of life's journey and adapt to change.

Communication becomes essential; a way to understand, connect, and foster growth. It is the art of communication that goes beyond words and creates an environment where partners can express their thoughts, fears and dreams.

Shared goals and hopes provide a beacon of the way forward. By providing a shared vision of the journey to success, people develop, transform and change as they grow. Every accomplishment, personal or shared, becomes a symbol of celebration and a testament to commitment to the relationship.

Recognition and happiness at this time will provide motivation for further growth and connection. is at the center of a supportive partnership; provides support, guidance and space for personal development. Partners become sources of motivation for each other, creating an environment that encourages self-discovery and expansion. This is the idea of continuous growth, adaptation and the courage to evolve.

Challenges are transformed into opportunities for learning and perseverance. Falling becomes a stepping stone that opens the way to deeper understanding and stronger connections. Consider participating in this dance of growth; a thoughtful pause to gauge the relationship. Now is the time to reflect on the implementation, revise it if necessary, and imagine a future of shared growth and harmony.

Seeking guidance together through mutual mentoring, mentoring, or professional discussion provides evidence of commitment to the union.

This is a recognition of those who thrive in an environment that encourages learning and broadens horizons.

Relationship development is based on commitment; an unconditional commitment to growing together. It is a commitment to supporting change, sustaining growth, and a love of relationships; each wire and each color represents a part of the unity; It is used primarily for the love of life and growth.

CONCLUSION

As we complete our exploration of the seven principles that make a successful marriage, it is clear that success in love is not just a place, but a continuous journey; It requires dedication, understanding and passion.

The meaning of these terms lies not only in their ideas but also in their application. It is the daily application of these principles that transforms relationships, giving them strength, depth and vulnerability.

Understanding the value of developing friendships, creating love maps, and cultivating mutual respect is the foundation of a strong partnership. Turning to each other during life's pressures, managing disagreements well, and supporting each other's dreams are the threads that have bind us together for a long time. Creating shared meaning, marked by shared and cherished moments, and fostering trust and commitment are fundamental to the sanctity of long-term relationships.

Following these principles requires not only understanding, but also small, consistent gestures that mean something, conversations that move the heart, and the satisfaction of growing individually and together.

When this journey ends, remember that applying these principles every day is what a successful relationship is all about. Think of these not as rigid rules but as signposts that will guide your relationship to a deeper, more intimate relationship; A partnership built from the ground up on trust, respect and unconditional love.

Let these principles be the guiding light that shows the power of using true meaning in love and friendship, pointing the way to a harmonious, lasting and harmonious relationship.

REVIEW

I truly appreciate your reaction.

Hello reader,

I hope this article will be useful to you. I'm reaching out to you as part of my ongoing journey to improve myself as a writer. Your response means a lot to me and I thank you for taking the time to share your thoughts.

Your experience as a reader means a lot, and I have worked hard to ensure that every page of this book leaves a positive impact. Your feedback can help me improve my writing and make it better and more relevant to you and others.

Would you take the time to share your thoughts and experiences with me? Your positive or negative feedback will help me understand your expectations better.

Please rest assured that your response will be treated with the utmost confidentiality and confidentiality.

Thank you for the importance of this journey. Your opinions are very important to me as I continue this process in order to serve you better.

Hello,

[Linda J. Lampley]

[Author]